Copyright 2020 by Omar Wilson -All rights reserved.

No part of this publication may be reproduced, distributed, or transmitted in any form or by any means, including photocopying, recording, or other electronic or mechanical methods, without the prior written permission of the publisher, except in the case of brief quotations embodied in reviews and certain other non-commercial uses permitted by copyright law.

This Book is provided with the sole purpose of providing relevant information on a specific topic for which every reasonable effort has been made to ensure that it is both accurate and reasonable. Nevertheless, by purchasing this Book you consent to the fact that the author, as well as the publisher, are in no way experts on the topics contained herein, regardless of any claims as such that may be made within. It is recommended that you always consult a professional prior to undertaking any of the advice or techniques discussed within. This is a legally binding declaration that is considered both valid and fair by both the Committee of Publishers Association and the American Bar Association and should be considered as legally binding within the United States.

CONTENTS

Introduction..4
Vegetarian Dishes...5
    Cheesy Eggplant Casserole 5
    Spinach & Mushroom Casserole 6
    Cheddar Carrot Risotto 7
    Green Risotto..8
    Bell Pepper Omelet 9
    Cheesy Stuffed Peppers...10
    Spicy Cabbage Soup 11
    Bok Choy Stir Fry 12
    Tomato Basil Soup...13
    Cheese & Broccoli Soup...14
Beef Recipes..15
    Beef & Spinach Casserole 15
    Bacon & Zucchini Casserole 16
    Taco Soup 17
    Beef & Broccoli Roast 18
    Chimichurri Skirt Steak 19
    Feta Burgers 20
Poultry Recipes...21
    Chicken & Artichoke Casserole 21
    Chicken Curry Casserole 22
    Asparagus Stuffed Chicken Breasts 23
    Creamy Spiced Chicken 24
    Ginger Chicken 25
    Grilled Chicken Skewers 26
    Buttery Garlic Chicken...27
    Cheesy Chicken & Broccoli 28
    Parmesan Chicken 29
    Chicken Milanese 30
Fish Recipes..31
    Celery & Grouper Casserole 31
    Lemon Butter Perch...32
    Shrimp & Broccoli..33
    Sea Bass & Spinach 34
    Chilled Lobster Soup 35
    Parmesan Shrimp Bake..36
    Roasted Mussels 37
    Curry Shrimp Soup..38
    Easy Lemon Butter Fish 39
    Fish Taco Bowls...40
    Parmesan Salmon & Asparagus 41
    Salmon Rice Bowls 42
    Scallops in a Bacon Sauce..43

- Creamy Salmon 44
- Butter Garlic Shrimp 45

Pork Recipes 46
- Pork Roast Casserole 46
- Kimchi Soup 47
- Broccoli & Bacon Casserole 48
- Bacon & Spinach Casserole 49
- Buttery Herb Pork Chops 50
- Parmesan Pork Chops & Asparagus 51
- Sesame Pork with Green Beans 52
- Kalua Pork & Cabbage 53
- Blue Cheese Pork Chops 54
- Pork Nachos 55
- Pork Burgers & Sriracha Mayonnaise 56

Side Dish Recipes 57
- Cheesy Asparagus 57
- Spicy Cauliflower 58
- Stuffed Mushrooms 59
- Lemon Spinach 60
- Red Cabbage Salad 61
- Garlic Mushrooms 62
- Braised Lemon Mushrooms 63

Introduction

The Ketogenic diet trend has already given us some amazing new ways to enjoy our food and we aren't going to lie, we are loving every minute of it! Is the Keto diet right for you?

A keto diet is well known for being a low carb diet, where the body produces ketones in the liver to be used as energy. It's referred to as many different names – ketogenic diet, low carb diet, low carb high fat, etc.

Ketosis is a natural process the body initiates to help us survive when food intake is low. During this state, we produce **ketones**, which are produced from the breakdown of fats in the liver.

The ketogenic diet is a miracle for your waist line and in general health, but it can be a nightmare to figure out what you can and can't cook. Some people think that it's only for snacks and salads, but that just isn't the case. In this ketogenic diet cookbook, you'll learn all about the dinner recipes that are sure to delight your taste buds and actually fill your stomach. Just because you 'There's no reason to deal with snacks for dinner when you have stuffed peppers, casseroles, and so much more to fill your plate!

Vegetarian Dishes
Cheesy Eggplant Casserole

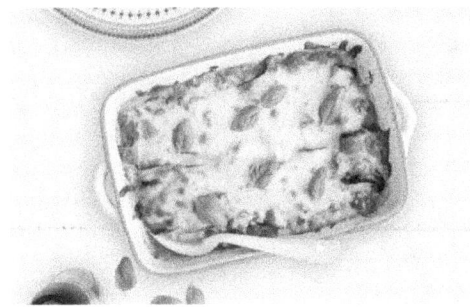

Serves: 2
Time: 35 Minutes
Calories: 496
Protein: 28 Grams
Fat: 39 Grams
Net Carbs: 8.1 Grams

Ingredients:
- 2 Eggplants
- 2 Tablespoons Olive Oil
- 1 ½ Cups Mozzarella Cheese, Grated
- 1 ½ Cups Marinara Sauce
- ½ Cup Parmesan Cheese
- Sea Salt to Taste
- 1 Tomato, Sliced
- Basil, Fresh & Chopped to Garnish
- Sea Salt & Black Pepper to Taste

Directions:
1. Start by heating your oven to 350, and then get outa baking tray. Line it with aluminum foil, and then grease it using a tablespoon of olive oil.
2. Slice your eggplant into thin slices, and then use a paper towel to get rid of excess moisture. Sprinkle your slices with salt, and then transfer them to a baking tray.
3. Bake your slices for three minutes before flipping them over, and then cook for another three minutes. Take the tray from the oven and set your slices aside without turning the oven off.
4. Take your casserole dish and grease it with another tablespoon of olive oil, and then add 1/3 of the marinara sauce, adding in your parmesan cheese. A layer of eggplants goes next, and then add in your mozzarella. Repeat until all ingredients except some parmesan are in your dish. Top with a layer of tomatoes and a final layer of parmesan cheese. Sprinkle with black pepper.
5. Fake for twenty minutes. Your cheese should turn a golden brown, and then take your casserole dish from the oven. Allow your dish to cool before topping with basil and serving warm.

Spinach & Mushroom Casserole

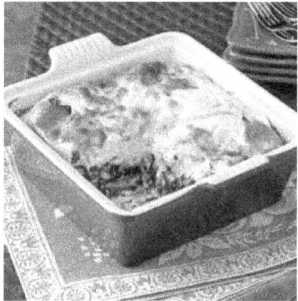

Serves: 6
Time: 1 Hour 30 Minutes
Calories: 149
Protein: 8.5 Grams
Fat: 9.4 Grams
Net Carbs: 3.9 Grams
Ingredients:

- 1 Celery Root, Large & Cubed
- 8 Ounces Baby Portobello Mushrooms, Quartered
- 1 Cup Vegetable Broth
- 3 Eggs
- 2 Cloves Garlic, Minced
- 2 Tablespoons Olive Oil
- 1 Onion, Diced
- 10 Ounces Spinach
- 1 ½ Cups Coconut Milk
- ½ Teaspoon Nutmeg
- Parsley, Fresh & Chopped Fine to Garnish
- Sea Salt & Black Pepper to Taste

Directions:

1. Start by heating your oven to 325, and then pulse your celery cubes in a food processor to form a "rice" before setting it to the side.
2. Get out a skillet, placing it over medium heat with oil, and cook your onion until tender. It should take about three minutes. Add in your garlic, cooking until fragrant which should take another minute. Add in your mushrooms and cook for another five minutes.
3. Add in spinach, cooking for another two minutes and adjust your seasonings if necessary.
4. Get out a bowl and beat your eggs with your nutmeg, milk and broth.
5. Get out a baking dish and place your rice in an even layer at the bottom before adding your vegetable on top. Pour in your egg mixture, and bake for fifty minutes. It should be golden, and then garnish with parsley before serving warm.

Cheddar Carrot Risotto

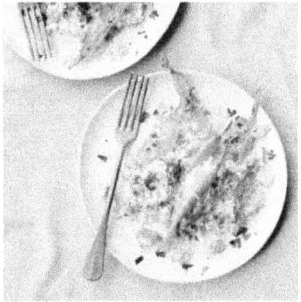

Serves: 2
Time: 25 Minutes
Calories: 342
Protein: 10.9 Grams
Fat: 25.8 Grams
Net Carbs: 7.3 Grams
Ingredients:
- 3 Teaspoons Jalapeno, Diced
- 1 Onion, Diced
- 2 Carrots, Large & Cubed
- 1 Lime, Juiced
- ½ Cup Cheddar Cheese, Grated
- 1 tablespoon Olive Oil
- ½ Teaspoon Chili Powder
- ½ Cup Vegetable Broth
- 1 Tablespoon Cilantro, Chopped
- ½ Avocado, Sliced
- Sea Salt & Black Pepper to Taste

Directions:
1. Pulse your carrot cubes in a food processor until you form a "rice". Set your carrot rice aside, and then get out a skillet. Place your skillet over medium heat, and add in your olive oil.
2. Once your oil is shimmering and hot add in your onion, cooking until soft. This should take about three minutes, and then stir in your rice. Add in your broth, lime juice, broth, chili powder and jalapenos. Season with salt and pepper, and then cook for ten minutes. Serve this topped with avocado.

Green Risotto

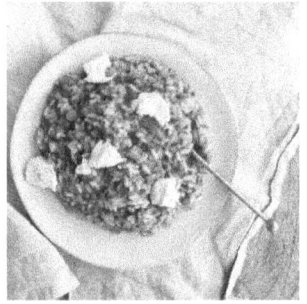

Serves: 2
Time: 30 Minutes
Calories: 191
Protein: 12.6 Grams
Fat: 10.7 Grams
Net Carbs: 7.9 Grams
Ingredients:
- 2 Scallions, Diced
- 1 Broccoli, Chopped into Florets
- 2 Eggs, Beaten
- ½ Cup Green Beans
- 1 Clove Garlic, Minced
- 1 Teaspoon Olive Oil
- ½ Cup Bell Pepper, Diced
- 1 Teaspoon Tamari Sauce
- ¼ Cup Reggiano Cheese, Grated
- Sea Salt & Black Pepper to Taste
- Parsley, Fresh & Chopped to Garnish

Directions:
1. Start by getting out a food processor and add your broccoli florets. Pulse until this forms a "rice". Set your rice to the side, and then get out a skillet.
2. Add your oil into the skillet, and then toss in your bell pepper, scallions and garlic. Cook for about three minutes until fragrant and tender, and then add in your broccoli rice. Cook for an additional two minutes.
3. Crack your eggs in, and then scramble them. Add in your tamari and green beans, and then adjust the seasoning as needed. Cook for a few more minutes until your green beans are softened.
4. Top with Parmesan, and then serve sprinkled with fresh parsley.

Bell Pepper Omelet

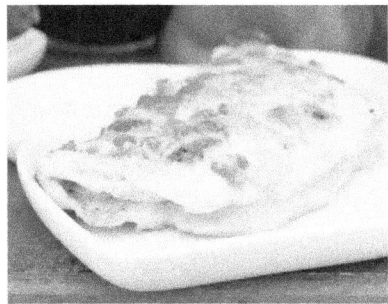

Serves: 1
Time: 15 Minutes
Calories: 415
Protein: 15.6 Grams
Fat: 33.1 Grams
Net Carbs: 6.1 Grams
Ingredients:
- 1 Teaspoon Olive Oil
- ½ Small Onion, Chopped
- 1 Bell Pepper, Chopped
- 1/3 Cup Tomatoes, Diced
- ¼ Cup Avocado, Sliced
- ¼ Teaspoon Thyme, Dry
- 2 Eggs, Large
- Sea Salt & Black Pepper to Taste

Directions:
1. Get out a skillet and heat your oil using medium heat, and then add in your bell pepper and onion. Cook for about five minutes. Your onion should have started to soften.
2. During this time beat your eggs lightly in a bowl and add in your salt, pepper and thyme. Pour your eggs over your vegetables, sprinkling your tomatoes on top.
3. In about three minutes, flip the omelet and then cook for another three minutes on that side.
4. Serve warm and topped with avocado slices.

Cheesy Stuffed Peppers

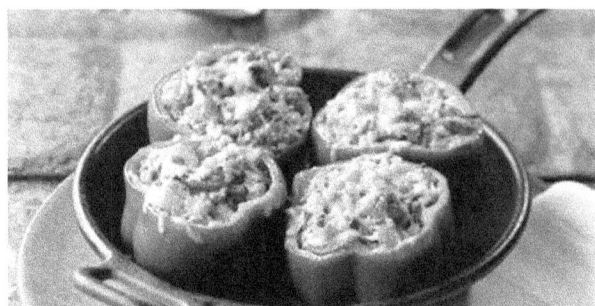

Serves: 4
Time: 35 Minutes
Calories: 243
Protein: 12 Grams
Fat: 15 Grams
Net Carbs: 5.6 Grams
Ingredients:
- 4 Bell Peppers, Seeded & Halved Lengthwise
- 4 Eggs, Large
- ½ Cup Cottage Cheese
- ½ Cup Queso Fresco
- ½ Cup Grana Padano, Grated
- 2 Cloves Garlic
- ½ Tomato
- ¼ Teaspoon Cilantro, Fresh & Chopped
- ¼ Cup Swiss Chard, Chopped

Directions:
1. Start by heating your oven to 350, and then grease a baking dish with cooking spray. Get out a food processor and blend together your cottage cheese, eggs, garlic, swiss chard, queso fresco, tomato and coriander.
2. Fill your peppers with the egg mixture, and then place them on a baking dish. Cover them with foil, baking for thirty to forty minutes.
3. Remove from oven, and sprinkle with Grana Padano, and then cook for another five minutes.

Spicy Cabbage Soup

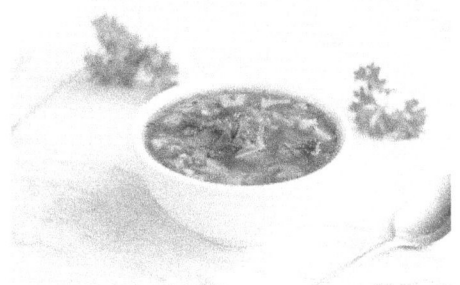

Serves: 6
Time: 20 Minutes
Calories: 94
Protein: 3.5 Grams
Fat: 6 Grams
Net Carbs: 5.3 Grams

Ingredients:
- 2 Cloves Garlic, Minced
- 1 Tablespoon Tallow
- 1 Onion, Chopped
- 1 Tomato, Grated
- ½ Head Cabbage, Sliced
- 1 Tablespoon Coconut Amino
- ¼ Cup Almonds, Ground
- Sea Salt to Taste
- 4 Cups Water
- Spicy Ground Paprika to Taste

Directions:
1. Start by getting on a frying pan and heating your tallow. Sauté your garlic and onion until golden brown and fragrant. Make sure to stir so that it doesn't burn. Add in your tomato and coconut aminos, stirring well.
2. add in your water, seasoning, ground almonds, cabbage, and then cover.
Allow it to simmer using medium heat for ten minutes, and then add in your paprika. Cook for another two to three minutes, and adjust your salt. Serve hot.

Bok Choy Stir Fry

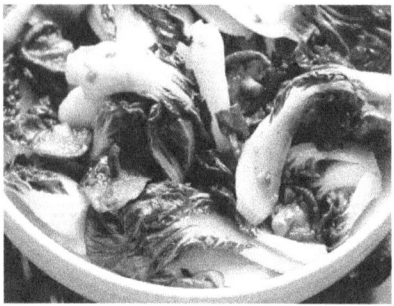

Serves: 2
Time: 25 Minutes
Calories: 134
Protein: 1 Gram
Fat: 14 Grams
Net Carbs: 2 Grams
Ingredients:
- 20 Ounces Bok Choy, Fresh
- 2 Tablespoons Olive Oil, Garlic infused
- 2 Green Onions, Chopped Fine
- 1 Tablespoon Oyster Sauce (Keto Friendly)
- 4 Tablespoons Water
- 1 Teaspoon Almond Flour
- Sea Salt to Taste

Directions:
1. Start by rinsing off your bok choy, and drain it well.
2. Heat your oil in a skillet, and sauté your onion and garlic together for three to four minutes. Make sure to stir well so that it doesn't burn. It should become fragrant and your onions tender.
3. Add your bok choy in, and cook for two to three minutes.
4. Get out a bowl and whisk your almond flour, water, salt and oyster sauce together. Pour this over your bok choy, and turn off the heat. Stir well, and allow it to sit for five minutes before serving warm.

Tomato Basil Soup

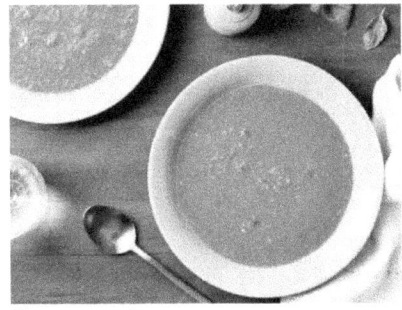

Serves: 4
Time: 20 Minutes
Calories: 239
Protein: 3 Grams
Fat: 22 Grams
Net Carbs: 7 Grams
Ingredients:
- 2 Ounces Cream Cheese
- 14.5 Ounces Diced Tomatoes, canned
- ¼ Cup Heavy Whipping Cream
- 4 Tablespoons Butter
- Sea Salt & Black Pepper to Taste
- ¼ Cup Basil Leaves, Fresh & Chopped

Directions:
1. Pour your tomatoes into a food processor, making sure not to drain their juices. Puree until it becomes smooth.
2. get out a medium saucepan, placing it over medium heat. Cook your tomatoes, heavy cream, cream cheese and butter together for ten minutes. Stir occasionally, and make sure it's mixed well.
3. add in your basil, seasoning with salt and pepper. Cook for another five minutes, and stir well. It should be completely smooth, and then use an immersion blender to blend well. Serve warm.

Cheese & Broccoli Soup

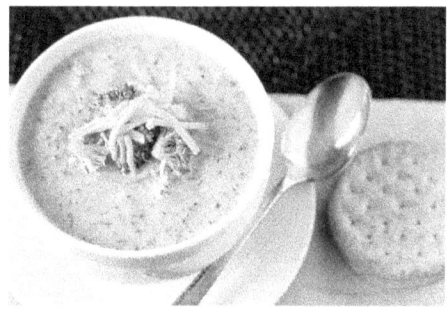

Serves: 4
Time: 25 Minutes
Calories: 383
Protein: 10 Grams
Fat: 37 Grams
Net Carbs: 4 Grams
Ingredients:
- 2 Tablespoons Butter
- 1 Cup Heavy Whipping Cream
- 1 Cup Broccoli Florets, Chopped Fine
- 1 Cup Vegetable Broth
- Sea Salt & Black Pepper to Taste
- 1 Cup Sharp Cheddar Cheese, Shredded, Some Reserved for Topping

Directions:
1. Start by getting out a medium saucepan, adding in your butter, and placing it over medium heat. Allow your butter to melt, and then add in your broccoli. Sauté until tender, which should take about five minutes.
2. Add in your vegetable broth and cream, stirring constantly. Season with salt and pepper, cooking for ten to fifteen minutes while stirring occasionally. Your soup should thicken. Turn the heat to low, and add in your shredded cheese. Reserve some for topping.
3. Serve warm and topped with remaining cheddar cheese.

Beef Recipes
Beef & Spinach Casserole

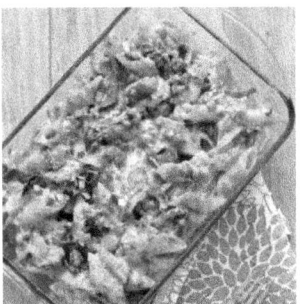

Serves: 4
Time: 55 Minutes
Calories: 484
Protein: 35 Grams
Fat: 36 Grams
Net Carbs: 1.5 Grams
Ingredients:
- 1 lb. Ground Beef
- Sea Salt & Black Pepper to Taste
- 1 Tomato, Sliced
- 2 Cups Baby Spinach
- 1 Cup Black Olives, Sliced
- 1 Tablespoon Cilantro, Fresh
- 8 Egg
- ½ Cup Parmesan Cheese, Grated

Directions:
1. Start by heating your oven to 350, and then get out a casserole dish. Add in your ground beef, sprinkling with salt and pepper, and then add in your lives, baby spinach, tomato, and then sprinkle with salt and cilantro.
2. Get out a bowl and whisk together your eggs until they turn frothy, adding in your grated cheese. Stir well. Season with salt and pepper if desired.
3. Pour this mixture into your casserole.
4. Bake for forty to forty-five minutes, and serve warm.

Bacon & Zucchini Casserole

Serves: 5
Time: 40 Minutes
Calories: 496
Protein: 19 Grams
Fat: 48 Grams
Net Carbs: 3.5 Grams
Ingredients:
- 1 Tablespoon Lard
- 1 lb. Bacon, Sliced into Strips
- 1 Spring Onion, Diced Fine
- 3 Zucchinis, Large
- Sea Salt & Black Pepper to Taste
- 6 Eggs
- ½ Container Feta Cheese, Crumbled

Directions:
1. Start by heating your oven to 350, and then get out a casserole dish. Grease your casserole dish with lard, and then put your bacon on the bottom. Top with green onions and then sliced zucchini rings. Season with salt and pepper.
2. Beat our eggs in a bowl, and then add in your salt and feta cheese, mixing well. Pour this mixture into your casserole dish next.
3. Cook for a half hour, and then slice and serve warm.

Taco Soup

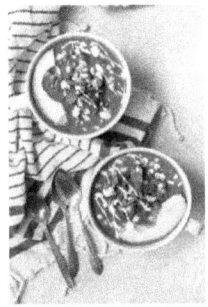

Serves: 4
Time: 4 Hours 15 Minutes
Calories: 422
Protein: 25 Grams
Fat: 33 Grams
Net Carbs: 5 Grams

Ingredients:
- 1 lb. Ground Beef
- Sea Salt & Black Pepper to Taste
- 2 Cups Beef Broth
- 10 Ounces Tomatoes, Diced & Canned
- 1 Tablespoon Taco Seasoning
- 8 Ounces Cream Cheese

Directions:
1. Preheat your slow cooker to low, and then get out a medium skillet. Sauté your ground beef over medium-high heat. Your meat should be browned, which will take about eight minutes. Season with salt and pepper.
2. Add your beef broth, tomatoes, taco seasoning, ground beef and cream cheese together in your slow cooker, cooking on low heat for four hours. You'll need to stir occasionally to keep it from burning.
3. Ladle for four bowls, and serve warm.

Beef & Broccoli Roast

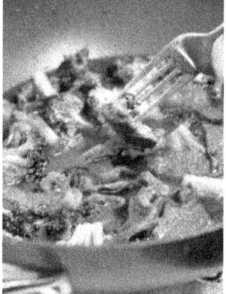

Serves: 2
Time: 4 Hours 40 Minutes
Calories: 806
Protein: 74 Grams
Fat: 49 Grams
Net Carbs: 12 Grams
Ingredients:
- 1 lb. Beef Chuck Roast
- Sea Salt & Black Pepper to Taste
- 16 Ounce Broccoli, Frozen
- 1 Teaspoon Toasted Sesame Oil
- ¼ Cup Soy Sauce
- ½ Cup Beef Broth + More as Needed

Directions:
1. Start by preheating your slow cooker to low, and then get out a cutting board. Place your roast on the cutting board, seasoning with salt and pepper. Slice thin, and then add it to the slower cooker.
2. Get out a small bowl, and mix your soy sauce, sesame oil and beef broth together, pouring it over the beef. Cook on low while covered for four hours, and then add in your frozen broccoli. Cook for a half hour more. Add additional beef broth if needed, and serve warm.

Chimichurri Skirt Steak

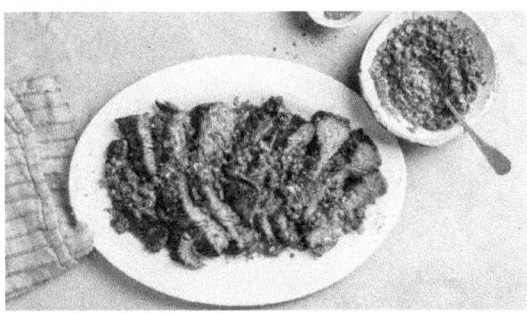

Serves: 2
Time: 8 Hours 20 Minutes
Calories: 718
Protein: 70 Grams
Fat: 46 Grams
Net Carbs: 4 Grams

Ingredients:
- Sea Salt & Black Pepper to Taste
- 1 Lime, Juiced
- ½ Cup Olive Oil
- 2 Tablespoons Apple Cider Vinegar
- 1 lb. Skirt Steak
- 2 Tablespoons Ghee
- ¼ Cup Chimichurri Sauce

Directions:
1. Start by getting out a small bowl, and mix your lime juice, olive oil, apple cider vinegar and soy sauce together.
2. Pour this mixture into a zipper top bag, and then add in your skirt steak. Marinate for at least eight hours.
3. Dry your steak with a paper towel, and then season with salt and pepper.
4. Get outa large skillet, and heat your ghee over high heat. Add in your steak, and sear for four minutes per side. It should be browned, and then place it on a cutting board. Allow your steak to rest for five minutes.
5. slice your steak against the grain, and then divide it between places, topping with chimichurri sauce.

Feta Burgers

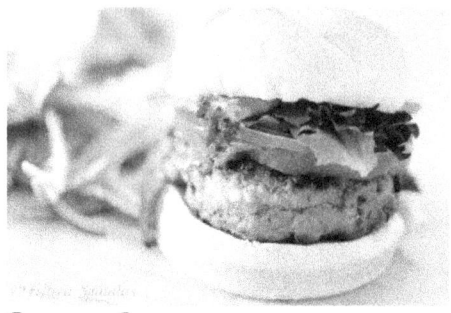

Serves: 2
Time: 20 Minutes
Calories: 607
Protein: 41 Grams
Fat: 48 Grams
Net Carbs: 2 Grams

Ingredients:
- 1 Tablespoon Ghee
- 1 Scallion, Sliced Thin
- 2 Tablespoons Mint Leaves, Fresh & Chopped Fine
- 1 Tablespoon Dijon Mustard
- Sea Salt & Black Pepper to Taste
- 12 Ounces Ground Beef & Ground Lamb Mixture
- 2 Ounces Feta Cheese, Crumbled

Directions:
1. Start by getting out a large bowl and mixing your mustard, scallion and mint leaves together. Add in your salt and pepper and mix well.
2. Add your ground beef and lamb into the bowl, mixing to form four patties.
3. Take your feta and press it into two of your patties with the other two on top. The cheese should be in the middle, and you'll need to seal the edges by pinching them closed.
4. Get out a medium skillet, placing it over medium heat, and add in your ghee. Once your ghee is hot, then add in your burgers, cooking for four to five minutes per side. Serve warm.

Poultry Recipes
Chicken & Artichoke Casserole

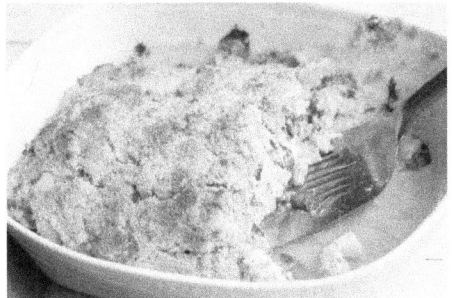

Serves: 4
Time: 35 Minutes
Calories: 101
Protein: 22 Grams
Fat: 29 Grams
Net Carbs: 2.5 Grams
Ingredients:
- 2 Tablespoons Butte
- 11 Ounces Artichoke Hearts, Drained
- 2 Green Onions, Chopped
- 1 Chicken Breast, Cubed
- ½ Cup White Wine, dry
- 1 Tablespoon Almond Flour
- ½ Cup Bone Broth
- ½ Cup Cream
- ¼ Teaspoon Tarragon Leaves
- 2 Tablespoons Parsley, Chopped for Garnish
- Sea Salt & Black Pepper to Taste

Directions:
1. Start by heating your oven to 350, and then get out a casserole dish. Grease it with butter. Cut your artichokes, and place them on the bottom of the casserole dish.
2. add your green onions and chicken cubes next.
3. Get out a bowl and combine your bone broth, wine, almond flour and cream, stirring well. Your almond flour should be completely dissolved, and then pour this mixture into your casserole dish as well.
4. Cook for twenty to twenty-five minutes, and serve warm.

Chicken Curry Casserole

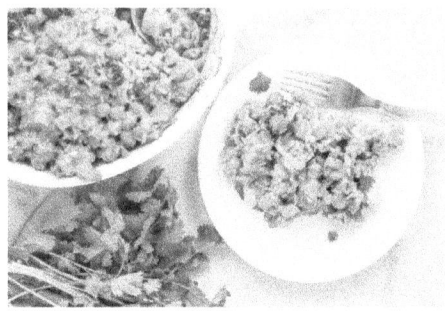

Serves: 4
Time: 35 Minutes
Calories: 186
Protein: 26 Grams
Fat: 8 Grams
Net Carbs: 4 Grams
Ingredients:
- 1 lb. Chicken Breast, Cubed
- 1 Tablespoon Chicken Fat
- 1 Onion, Sliced Fine
- 1 Carrot
- 2 Teaspoons Curry Powder
- 1 Pinch Saffron
- ½ Cup Wine
- ½ Cup Bone Broth
- 1 Tablespoon Coriander, Fresh
- Sea Salt to Taste

Directions:
1. Start by cutting your chicken breasts into cubes, and then heat your chicken fat, sautéing your onion over medium-high heat.
2. Add in your chicken cubes, browning them on all sides. Stir well. This should take two to three minutes. Sprinkle with saffron and curry before adding n your carrot. Stir well, and then pour in your bone broth and wine. Stir again, and season with salt. Cover and allow it to simmer for twenty minutes.
3. sprinkle with coriander leaves, and serve warm.

Asparagus Stuffed Chicken Breasts

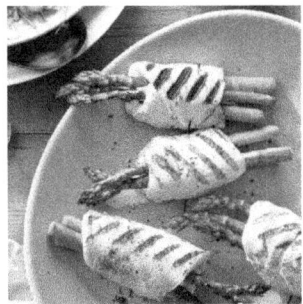

Serves: 4
Time: 45 Minutes
Calories: 236
Protein: 32 Grams
Fat: 30 Grams
Net Carbs: 1.8 Grams

Ingredients:

- 2 Chicken Breasts Halves, Skinless & Boneless
- 8 Asparagus Spears, Trimmed
- ½ Cup Parmesan Cheese, Shredded
- ¼ Cup Ground Almonds
- Sea Salt & Black Pepper to Taste

Directions:

1. Start by heating your oven to 375, and then grease a baking dish. Set your baking dish to the side.
2. Place each chicken breast between freezer bags before putting it on a solid surface, flattening some before sprinkling with salt and pepper. Lay four spears in the center of each, and then spread ¼ cup of parmesan over the asparagus. Repeat with your other breast, and then roll well.
3. Put your rolls in the baking dish, making sure that the seam is facing downward. Sprinkle with two tablespoons of ground almonds for each one. Bake for twenty-five to thirty minutes, and allow to cool for ten minutes before serving warm.

Creamy Spiced Chicken

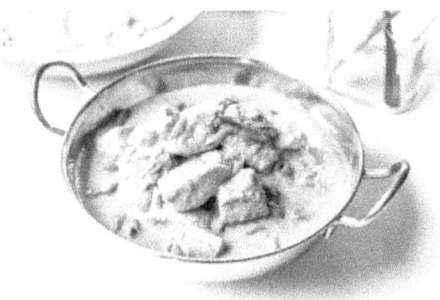

Serves: 8
Time: 1 Hour
Calories: 420
Protein: 31 Grams
Fat: 32 Grams
Net Carbs: 1.8 Grams

Ingredients:
- 2 teaspoons Chicken Fat
- 1 Whole Chicken, Cut Up
- ½ Cup Ground Almonds
- ½ Teaspoon Onion Powder
- ¼ Teaspoon Cayenne Pepper
- 1/8 Teaspoon Ground Ginger
- ½ Teaspoon Garlic Powder
- 1/3 Cup Yogurt, Plain

Directions:
1. Start by heating your oven to 360, and then get out a baking tray. Grease your bacon tray with the chicken fat before setting it o the side. Cut your chicken into large parts, and then rinse it and pat it dry.
2. Get out a large bowl and combine your onion powder, garlic powder, ground almonds, cayenne pepper and ginger together. Dip your chicken into the yogurt, and then roll them into the almond mixture. This will make your "breading".
3. Place your chicken in the baking dish, and then bake for forty-five to fifty minutes. Do not cover your chicken.

Ginger Chicken

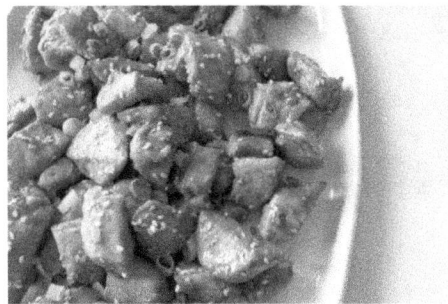

Serves: 6
Time: 45 Minutes
Calories: 468
Protein: 49 Grams
Fat: 28 Grams
Net Carbs: 0.8 Grams

Ingredients:
- ½ Whole Chicken, Chopped
- Sea Salt to Taste
- ¼ Cup Ginger, Grated
- 1 Tablespoon Coconut Aminos
- 2 Tablespoon Red Wine
- ½ Cup Sesame Oil
- 2 Tablespoons Spring Onion, Chopped

Directions:
1. Rub your chicken down with salt, and then place it in a bot that's been fitted with a steamer basket over water. Steam your chicken using medium-high heat for a half hour. Your chicken should be cooked all the way through. Drain your chicken, and then reserve ¼ a cup of the "soup".
2. In a frying skillet heat your ginger, sesame, coconut aminos, reserved soup and wine together. Cook for two minutes, and don't forget to stir.
3. Remove the chicken, and pour your sauce over it, garnishing with spring onions and serving warm.

Grilled Chicken Skewers

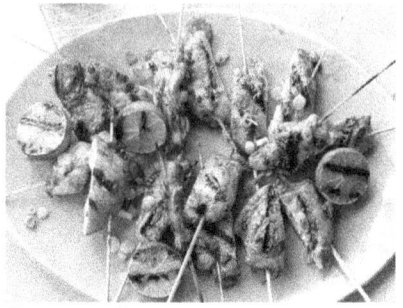

Serves: 2
Time: 1 Hour 25 Minutes
Calories: 586
Protein: 75 Grams
Fat: 29 Grams
Net Carbs: 5 Grams

Ingredients:
- 1 lb. Chicken Breast, Boneless, Skinless & Chunked
- 3 Tablespoons Coconut Aminos, Divided
- ½ Teaspoon Sriracha Sauce + ¼ Teaspoon
- 3 Tablespoons Toasted Sesame Oil, Divided
- Ghee for Oiling
- 2 Tablespoons Peanut Butter
- Sea Salt & Black Pepper to Taste

Directions:
1. Get out a zipper top bag, and combine your chicken, coconut aminos, ½ teaspoon Sriracha sauce, and two teaspoons of sesame oil before sealing it. Allow it to marinate for an hour or overnight. Remember that you'll need to soak your skewers for a half hour before using them.
2. preheat your grill, oiling it with ghee if necessary. Thread your chicken onto your skewers, and cook for ten to fifteen minutes on low heat. You'll need to flip your skewers halfway through.
3. Mix your peanut dipping sauce by stirring together a tablespoon of coconut aminos, ¼ teaspoon Sriracha sauce, a teaspoon of sesame oil and peanut butter. Mix well and season with salt and pepper. Serve your chicken with peanut sauce.

Buttery Garlic Chicken

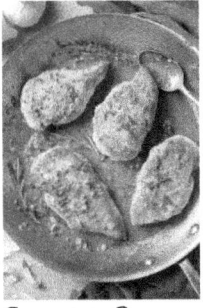

Serves: 2
Time: 45 Minutes
Calories: 642
Protein: 57 Grams
Fat: 45 Grams
Net Carbs: 2 Grams
Ingredients:
- 2 Cloves Garlic, Minced
- ¼ Cup Parmesan Cheese, Grated
- 1 Tablespoon Italian Seasoning
- Sea Salt & Black Pepper to Taste
- 4 Tablespoons Butter
- 2 Chicken Breasts, Boneless & Skinless
- 2 Tablespoons Ghee, Melted

Directions:
1. Start by heating your oven to 375, and then get out a baking dish. Pat your chicken dry and then season it with Italian seasoning, salt and pepper. Place them in the baking dish.
2. Get out a medium skillet, placing it over medium heat and melt your butter. Add in your garlic, and cook for five minutes. Make sure to stir so that your garlic doesn't burn. It should be lightly browned and fragrant. Remove the mixture from heat, pouring it over your chicken.
3. Roast your chicken for thirty to thirty-five minutes, and then sprinkle with parmesan. Allow it to rest for five minutes before serving.

Cheesy Chicken & Broccoli

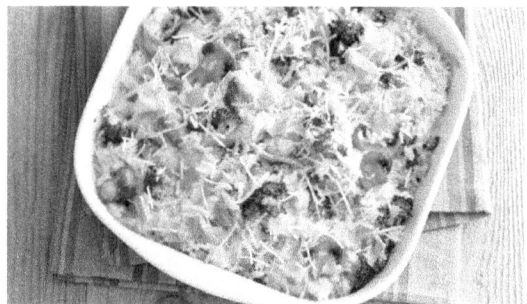

Serves: 2
Time: 1 Hour 10 Minutes
Calories: 935
Protein: 75 Grams
Fat: 66 Grams
Net Carbs: 8 Grams

Ingredients:
- 2 Chicken Breasts, Boneless & Skinless
- Sea Salt & Black Pepper to Taste
- 4 Bacon Slices
- 2 Tablespoons Ghee
- 2 Cups Broccoli Florets, Frozen & Thawed
- ½ Cup Cheddar Cheese, Shredded
- 6 Ounces Cream Cheese, Room Temperature

Directions:
1. Start by heating your oven to 375.
2. Get out a baking dish, and coat it with ghee. Pat your chicken dry before seasoning it with salt and pepper. Place your chicken along with your bacon slices in your baking dish, cooking for twenty-five minutes.
3. Transfer your chicken to a chopping board, and shred it. Season with salt and pepper again if necessary. Place your bacon on a plate that's been lined with paper towels. Crumble your bacon once it crisps up from sitting.
4. Get out a medium bowl, and combine your shredded chicken, cream cheeses, broccoli and half of your bacon. Transfer this mixture to your baking dish, topping with cheese and your remaining bacon.
5. Bake until your cheese is browned and bubbling, which should take about thirty-five minutes. Serve warm.

Parmesan Chicken

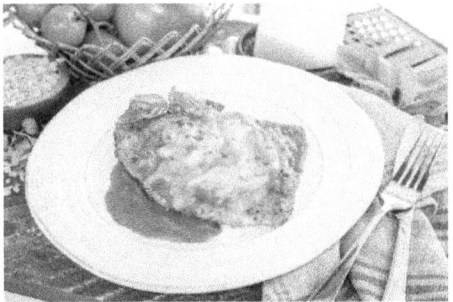

Serves: 2 **Time:** 25 Minutes
Calories: 850
Protein: 60 Grams
Fat: 67 Grams
Net Carbs: 2 Grams

Ingredients:
- 2 Tablespoons Ghee
- 2 Chicken Breasts, Boneless & Skinless / ½ Cup Mayonnaise
- 1 Tablespoon Italian Seasoning
- ¼ Cup Parmesan Cheese, Grated
- Sea Salt & Black Pepper to Taste
- ¼ Cup Pork Rinds, Crushed

Directions:
1. Start by heating your oven to 425, and then get out a baking dish.
2. Coat your baking dish with ghee, and then pat your chicken dry before seasoning it with salt and pepper. Place your chicken in your dish, and then get out a small bowl.
3. In your bowl mix your parmesan, Italian seasoning and mayonnaise, slathering this mixture over your chicken. Sprinkle your pork rinds over this mixture, and bake for twenty minutes. The top should be browned, and serve warm.

Chicken Milanese

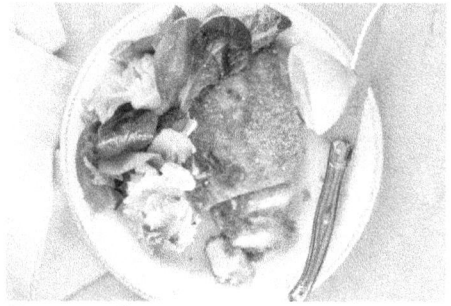

Serves: 2
Time: 20 Minutes
Calories: 604
Protein: 65 Grams
Fat: 29 Grams
Net Carbs: 7 Grams

Ingredients:
- 1 Teaspoon Cayenne Pepper
- ½ Cup Coconut Flour
- 2 Chicken Breasts, Boneless & Skinless
- Sea Salt & Black Pepper to Taste
- 1 Egg, Beaten Lightly
- ½ Cup Pork Rinds, Crushed
- 2 Tablespoons Olive Oil

Directions:
1. Start by getting out ap lace and place your coconut flour, salt, pepper, and cayenne pepper in it. Mix well.
2. Get out a bowl and crack your egg in it. Beat it with a fork until it's whisked well.
3. get out another plate, and place your crushed pork rinds on it. Get out a skillet, and place it over medium-high heat, heating up your olive oil.
4. Dredge your chicken through the coconut flour on both sides before dipping it into your egg and coating it with pork rinds. Place it in the skillet, and cook for three to five minutes per side. It should be crispy and browned. Serve warm.

Fish Recipes
Celery & Grouper Casserole

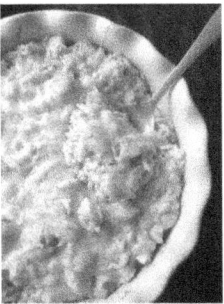

Serves: 8
Time: 25 Minutes
Calories: 371
Protein: 23 Grams
Fat: 29 Grams
Net Carbs: 1.9 Grams
Ingredients:
- 3 ½ lbs. Grouper Fish
- 1 ½ lbs. Celery, Fresh & Chopped
- 1 Cup Olive Oil
- ½ Cup White Wine
- Sea Salt & Black Pepper to Taste
- 1 Lemon, Juiced

Directions:
1. Season your grouper with salt and pepper, and then rinse and clean your celery. Chop your celery fine, and then place your celery in a large saucepan. Place your fish slices over the celery, and pour the olive oil, lemon juice and wine. Cook over high heat until it boils.
2. Reduce the heat to medium, cover and cook for five to six minutes.
3. Taste and adjust your salt and pepper as necessary and serve warm.

Lemon Butter Perch

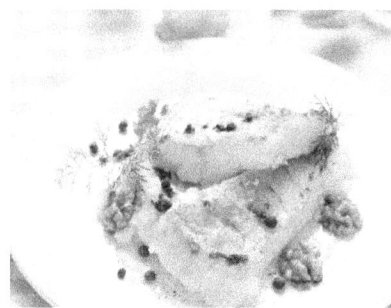

Serves: 4
Time: 30 Minutes
Calories: 297
Protein: 47 Grams
Fat: 10 Grams
Net Carbs: 0 Grams
Ingredients:
- 3 Tablespoons Olive Oil
- 2 tablespoons Butter, Unsalted
- 1 Lemon, Sliced
- 2 Tablespoons Lemon Juice
- 1 Lemon, Zested
- 6 Perch Fillets
- Sea Salt & Black Pepper to Taste
- 2 Tablespoons Parsley, Fresh & Chopped Fine

Directions:
1. Start by heating your oven to 360, and then grease a baking dish with olive oil. Mix your olive oil, lemon juice, lemon zest and butter in a bowl, making sure to stir well.
2. season your fish fillets with salt and pepper before arranging them on a baking dish, pouring your butter mixture evenly over your fillets. Cover with lemon slices, and then bake for fifteen to twenty minutes. Serve warm with chopped parsley.

Shrimp & Broccoli

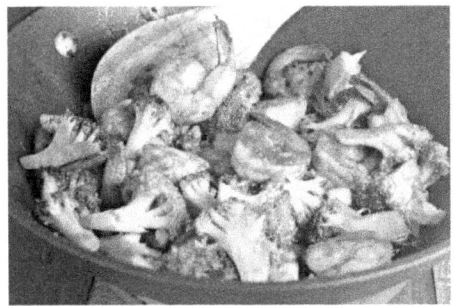

Serves: 4
Time: 30 Minutes
Calories: 220
Protein: 27 Grams
Fat: 10 Grams
Net Carbs: 6.3 Grams

Ingredients:
- 2 Tablespoons Sesame Oil
- 4 Cloves Garlic, Minced
- 1 Cup Water
- 2 Teaspoons Ginger Root, Fresh & Grated
- 2 Tablespoons Coconut Aminos
- 2 Cups Broccoli Florets, Fresh
- 1 ½ lbs. Shrimp, Peeled & Deveined
- Lemon Wedges for Garnish

Directions:
1. Start by heating up a large skillet or wok using medium-high heat, and then add in your garlic. Allow your garlic to cook for three to four minutes before reducing the heat to low. Add in your ginger, coconut aminos and water. Bring this mixture to a boil.
2. Cook until your shrimp turn pink, which should take three to four minutes. Add in your broccoli, cooking for an additional ten minutes. Serve hot with lemon wedges to garnish.

Sea Bass & Spinach

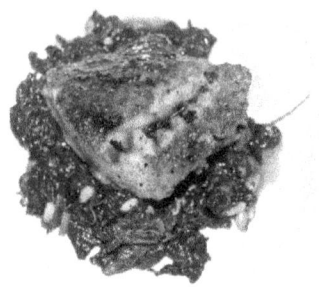

Serves: 6
Time: 25 Minutes
Calories: 312
Protein: 34 Grams
Fat: 15 Grams
Net Carbs: 4 Grams
Ingredients:
- ½ Cup White Wine
- Sea Salt & Black Pepper to Taste
- ¼ Cup Olive Oil
- 1 Onion, Chopped Fine
- 1 Green Onion, Sliced
- 2 Cloves Garlic
- 2 Lemons, Juiced & Zested
- 1 lb. Spinach, Fresh
- ½ Cup Water
- 4 Sea Bass Fillets
- Lemon Slices for Garnish
- 1/3 Bunch Dill for Garnish
- 1 Tablespoon Olive Oil to Serve

Directions:
1. Start by heating your olive oil in a large skillet, placing it over high heat.
2. Chop your onion and green onion, placing it in your pan and sauté with garlic for three to four minutes. It should be lightly browned and fragrant. Season with salt and pepper, and cook for another minute. Make sure that you stir to avoid burning.
3. Pour in your wine, allowing it to sit for one to two minutes. This should give it time to evaporate, and then add in your lemon juice and lemon zest, stirring well.
4. Add in your chopped spinach and water, and then stir well. Allow it to cook for five more minutes.
5. Add in your fish fillets, and then season with olive oil and pepper. Cover, cooking for four minutes using medium heat.
6. Serve hot with dill and olive oil.

Chilled Lobster Soup

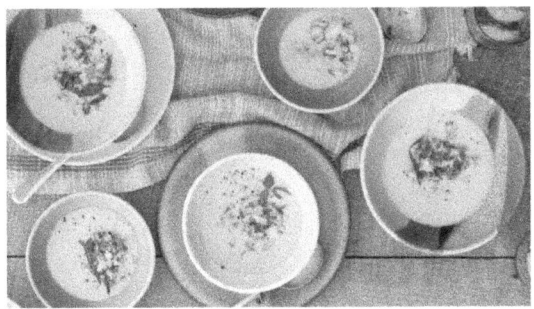

Serves: 4
Time: 15 Minutes
Calories: 255
Protein: 38 Grams
Fat: 9 Grams
Net Carbs: 1.5 Grams
Ingredients:
- 1 Cup Water
- ¼ Cup Ground Almonds
- 1 Cup Red Wine
- 2 Teaspoons Cardamom Seeds
- Sea Salt & Black Pepper to Taste
- 1 Large Tomato, Grated
- 2 Tablespoons Olive Oil
- 1 Tablespoon Chives, Fresh & Chopped
- 30 Ounces Lobster Meat, Canned

Directions:
1. Start by adding in your lobster meat into a pot, and drizzle with olive oil. Season with salt and pepper before adding in your chopped chives and cardamom. Add in your grated tomato, water and red wine.
2. cook for six to seven minutes over medium heat before adding in your ground almonds. Make sure to stir well, and adjust seasoning as necessary. Serve warm or chilled.

Parmesan Shrimp Bake

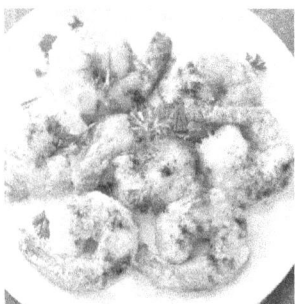

Serves: 6
Time: 30 Minutes
Calories: 295
Protein: 26 Grams
Fat: 19 Grams
Net Carbs: 3.2 Grams
Ingredients:
- 2 lbs. Shrimp, Peeled
- Sea Salt & Black Pepper to Taste
- 1 Lemon Juice, Zested & Juiced
- 1/3 Cup Olive Oil
- 2 Tablespoons Oregano, Fresh & Chopped
- ¼ Cup Almonds, Ground
- 4 Cloves Garlic
- ½ Cup Parmesan, Grated
- Pinch Chili Flakes
- 1 Bunch Parsley, Fresh & Chopped
- 1 Tablespoon Basil, Fresh
- Lemon Wedges for Garnish

Directions:
1. Start by heating your oven to 400, and then get out a bowl. Combine your lemon zest, lemon juice, salt, pepper, olive oil and shrimp together, stirring well. Add in your oregano, and stir again before setting it to the side.
2. Get out a blender and mix together your ground almonds, parmesan, garlic, chili flakes, oregano, and lemon zest. Blend until combined well. Add this mixture you're your shrimp bowl, stirring gently.
3. Lay your shrimp out on a baking dish, baking for ten to twelve minutes. Serve with lemon wedges while still warm.

Roasted Mussels

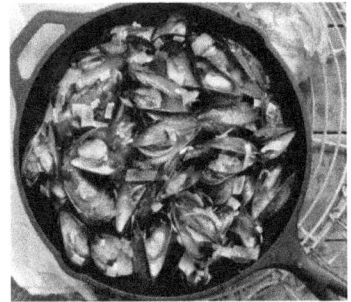

Serves; 6
Time: 40 Minutes
Calories: 355
Protein: 23 Grams
Fat: 25 Grams
Net Carbs: 6 Grams

Ingredients:
- 2 lbs. Mussels
- ¾ Cup Water
- Coarse Salt for Baking Dish
- 1/3 Cup Olive Oil
- ¾ Cup Ground Almond
- 2 Cloves Garlic, Chopped
- 4 Tablespoons Parmesan, Grated
- 1 Bunch Parsley, Chopped Fine
- 1 Teaspoon Oregano, Fresh
- Sea Salt to Taste

Directions:
1. Start by heating your oven to 450, and then rinse and clean your mussels using cold water.
2. get out a large pot, and then heat your water, adding in your mussels. Bring it to a boil and cover, cooking for five to six minutes.
3. Use a pierced ladle to transfer them to a bowl, but reserve the cooking liquid. Remove half of the shell, and allow for the other half to hold the mussel.
4. Get out a baking pan, and sprinkle with thick salt, laying your mussels over it, and pour in some liquid.
5. Get out a bowl and mix together your olive oil, ground almonds, garlic, parsley, oregano, salt and parmesan, dividing it over the mussels evenly.
6. Bake for fifteen minutes before serving hot.

Curry Shrimp Soup

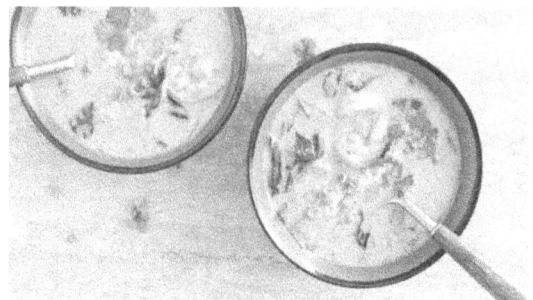

Serves: 4 **Time:** 2 Hours 20 Minutes
Calories: 269
Protein: 16 Grams **Fat:** 21 Grams
Net Carbs: 18 Grams

Ingredients:
- 8 Ounces Water
- 13.4 Ounces Full Fat Coconut Milk, Canned & Unsweetened
- 2 Cups Riced Cauliflower
- 2 Tablespoons Red Curry Paste
- 2 Tablespoons Cilantro, Fresh & Chopped
- Sea Salt & Black Pepper to Taste
- 1 Cup Shrimp, Cooked, Peeled & Deveined

Directions:
1. Start by preheating your slow cooker to high.
2. Add in your coconut milk, cauliflower rice, water, red curry paste, and a tablespoon of your fresh, chopped cilantro. Season with salt and pepper, and stir well. Cover, cooking for two hours on high heat.
3. Season your shrimp with slat and pepper before adding them in, stirring well. Allow it to cook for another fifteen minutes, and top with your remaining cilantro before serving warm.

Easy Lemon Butter Fish

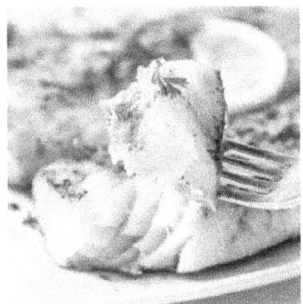

Serves: 2
Time: 30 Minutes
Calories: 299
Protein: 16 Grams
Fat: 26 Grams
Net Carbs: 3 Grams
Ingredients:
- 4 Tablespoons Butter
- 2 Tilapia Fillets, 5 Ounces Each
- Pink Himalayan Sea Salt, Fine
- Ground Black Pepper to Taste
- 3 Cloves Garlic, Minced
- 2 Tablespoons Capers, Rinsed & Chopped
- 1 Lemon, Zested & Juiced

Directions:
1. Start by heating your oven to 400, and then get out an eight inch baking dish. Coat your dish with butter, and then take out your fish.
2. pat your fish with paper towels to dry it, and then season both sides with slat and pepper before placing them in your buttered dish.
3. Take out a medium skillet, and then place it over medium heat. Melt your butter, and add in garlic. Cook for three to five minutes. Your garlic should be fragrant and browned slightly, but be careful to make sure that you don't burn it.
4. Pour your garlic infused butter into a bowl, adding in two tablespoons of lemon juice and lemon zest. Mix well, and pour this mixture over your fish.
5. Sprinkle your capers around the fish. Bake for twelve to fifteen minutes, and serve warm. Your fish should be cooked through and flaky.

Fish Taco Bowls

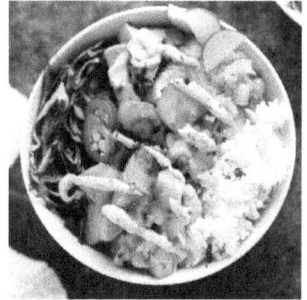

Serves: 2
Time: 25 Minutes
Calories: 315
Protein: 16 Grams
Fat: 24 Grams
Net Carbs: 5 Grams

Ingredients:
- 2 White Fish Fillets, 5 Ounces Each
- 1 Tablespoon Olive Oil
- 4 Teaspoons Tajin Seasoning Salt, Divided
- 2 cups Coleslaw Cabbage Mix, Pre-Sliced
- 1 Avocado, Mashed
- Sea Salt & Black Pepper to Taste
- 1 Tablespoon Red Pepper Miso Mayo + More for Serving

Directions:
1. Start by heating your oven to 425, and then line a baking sheet using foil.
2. rub your white fish down with your olive oil, coating it with your tajin seasoning salt, using only two teaspoons. Place it on a prepared pan before baking for fifteen minutes. Your fish should become opaque when pierced using a fork. Allow your fish to cool on a cooling rack for four minutes.
3. While your fish cools, get out a medium bowl and mix your mayo sauce and coleslaw together. Add in your avocado and remaining tajin seasoning salt. Mix and season with salt and pepper. Divide between bowls, and top with shredded fish before drizzling more mayo sauce on to before serving.

Parmesan Salmon & Asparagus

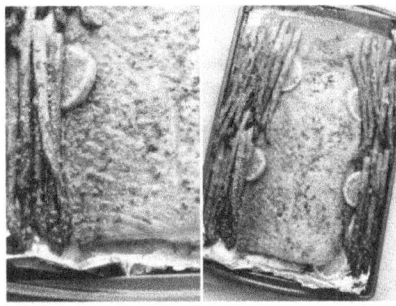

Serves: 2
Time: 25 Minutes
Calories: 434
Protein: 42 Grams
Fat: 26 Grams
Net Carbs: 6 Grams

Ingredients:
- 2 Salmon Fillets, 6 Ounces Each & Skin On
- Sea Salt & Black Pepper to Taste
- 3 Tablespoons Butter
- ¼ Cup Parmesan Cheese, Grated
- 2 Cloves Garlic, Minced
- 1 lb. Asparagus, Fresh & Trimmed

Directions:
1. Start by heating your oven to 400, and then get out a baking sheet. Line your baking sheet with foil before placing it to the side.
2. Pat your salmon down with a paper towel so that it's dry, and then season with salt and pepper.
3. Put your salmon your baking pan, arranging your asparagus around it.
4. Get out a saucepan, placing it over medium heat to melt your butter. Once your butter has melted add in your garlic, and stir. Cook until your garlic is lightly browned and fragrant. This should take about three minutes. Drizzle this butter over your asparagus and salmon.
5. Top with parmesan before baking of twelve minutes. Broil for the last three minutes, and serve warm.

Salmon Rice Bowls

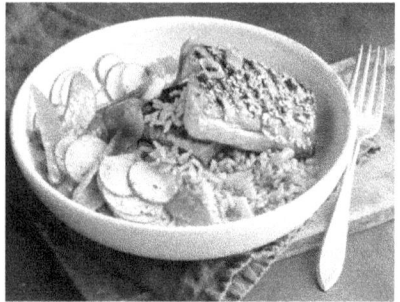

Serves: 2
Time: 50 Minutes
Calories: 328
Protein: 36 Grams
Fat: 18 Grams
Net Carbs: 5 Grams

Ingredients:
- 2 Salmon Fillets, 6 Ounces Each & Skin On
- 4 Tablespoons Soy Sauce, Divided
- 2 Small Persian Cucumbers
- 1 Tablespoon Ghee
- 1 Avocado, Diced
- 8 Ounces Shirataki Rice
- Sea Salt & Black Pepper to Taste

Directions:
1. Start by getting out an eight inch baking dish, and add three tablespoons of soy sauce to it. Placing your salmon in. allow it to marinate for thirty minutes.
2. While your fish is marinating, slicing your cucumbers thin before placing them in a small bowl, adding in a tablespoon of soy sauce, allowing them to marinate as well.
3. Get out a medium skillet and place it over medium heat. Add in your ghee, and allow it to melt. Add your salmon in, making sur that it's skin side down. Pour some of the marinade over it, and sear for three to four minutes per side.
4. Get out a large saucepan, and then cook your rice per package instructions. Rinse your rice in a colander.
5. Transfer your rice to a dry pan, and roast until opaque and dry. Season your avocado with salt and pepper, and then plate your salmon fillets to cut them.
6. Divide all ingredients between bowls before serving.

Scallops in a Bacon Sauce

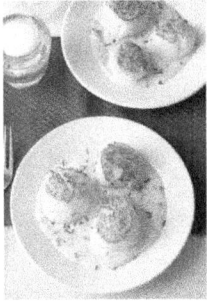

Serves: 2
Time: 25 Minutes
Calories: 782
Protein: 24 Grams
Fat: 73 Grams
Net Carbs: 10 Grams
Ingredients:
- 4 Bacon Slices
- 1 Cup Heavy Whipping Cream
- ¼ Cup Parmesan Cheese, Grated
- 1 Tablespoon Butter
- Sea Salt & Black Pepper to Taste
- 1 Tablespoon Ghee
- 8 Sea Scallops, Large, Rinsed & Patted Dry

Directions:
1. Get out a medium skillet and place it over medium-high heat, cooking your bacon on both sides until it turns crispy. This will take about eight minutes, and then line a plate with paper towels. Place your bacon on it so that it can drain.
2. lower your heat to medium before adding in your butter, cream, and parmesan. Season with a pinch of salt and pepper before reducing your heat further to low. Cook, and stir constantly so that your sauce thickens and reduces by half without burning. This will take about ten minutes.
3. Get out a different skillet placing it over medium-high heat, adding in your ghee. Cook it until it sizzles.
4. Get out your scallops and sprinkle with salt and pepper before adding them to your hot skillet, cooking for a minute per side. You have to make sure you don't crowd your scallops, so cook int wo batches if necessary. They should be golden on both sides.
5. Drain your scallops on a plate lined in paper towels, and then divide them between places. Top with sauce before serving warm.

Creamy Salmon

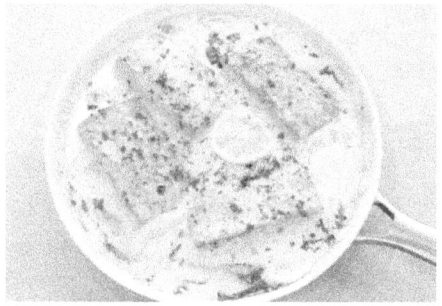

Serves: 2
Time: 20 Minutes
Calories: 510
Protein: 33 Grams
Fat: 41 Grams
Net Carbs: 2 Grams

Ingredients:
- 2 Tablespoons Ghee, Melted
- 2 Salmon Fillets, 6 Ounces Each & Skin On
- Sea Salt & Black Pepper to Taste
- ¼ Cup Mayonnaise
- 2 Tablespoons Dill, Fresh & Minced
- 1 Tablespoon Dijon Mustard
- Pinch Garlic Powder

Directions:
1. Start by heating your oven to 450, and then get out a nine by thirteen inch pan. Grease it with your ghee.
2. Take your salmon and pat it down with paper towels to dry it. Season with salt and pepper before placing it in your baking dish.
3. Get out a small bowl and mix your mustard, dill, garlic powder and mayonnaise.
4. Slather this sauce on top of your fillets, and then bake for seven to nine minutes depending on preference. Serve warm.

Butter Garlic Shrimp

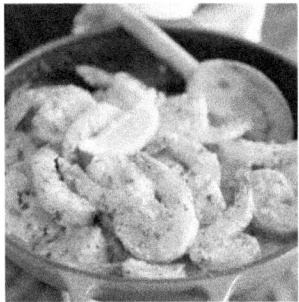

Serves: 2
Time: 25 Minutes
Calories: 329
Protein: 32 Grams
Fat: 20 Grams
Net Carbs: 4 Grams

Ingredients:
- 3 Tablespoons Butter
- ½ lb. Shrimp, Peeled & Deveined
- 3 Cloves Garlic, Crushed
- 1 Lemon, Halved
- ¼ Teaspoon Red Pepper Flakes
- Sea Salt & Black Pepper to Taste

Directions:
1. Start by heating your oven to 425, and then put your butter in an eight inch baking dish. Place it in the oven to preheat.
2. Season your shrimp with salt and pepper, and then slice your half a lemon in thin slices. Cut your other in half into two different wedges.
3. add your shrimp, butter and garlic into the dish with your shrimp. Make sure your shrimp is placed in a single layer, and then sprinkle with red pepper flakes.
4. Bake for fifteen minutes, but stir at the seven minute mark.
5. Remove from the oven, and squeeze your lemon wedges over your shrimp before serving.

Pork Recipes
Pork Roast Casserole

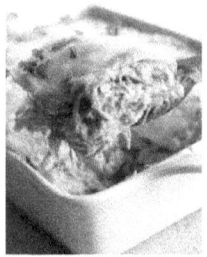

Serves: 5
Time: 1 Hour 10 Minutes
Calories: 549
Protein: 43.5 Grams
Fat: 40 Grams
Net Carbs: 1.9 Grams
Ingredients:
- 2 Tablespoon Butter
- 2 lbs. Pork Roast
- 1 Green Onion, Chopped
- 1 Tablespoon Almond Flour
- ½ Cup White Wine
- 1 Cup Bone Broth
- ½ Cup Cream
- 3 Tarragon Sprigs, Fresh
- 3 Slices cheddar Cheese
- sea Salt & Black Pepper to Taste

Directions:
1. Heat your butter in a skillet over medium heat, and then brown your roast for five to six minutes. Add in your green onion, and then pour the wine in. allow it to simmer for two to three minutes.
2. Place everything into a casserole dish, and then add in your wine. Season with salt and pepper and cook, covered with your bone broth for thirty to thirty-five minutes. Add in the cream and chopped tarragon, stirring gently. Place your cheddar slices on top and cook for another fifteen minutes. Serve warm.

Kimchi Soup

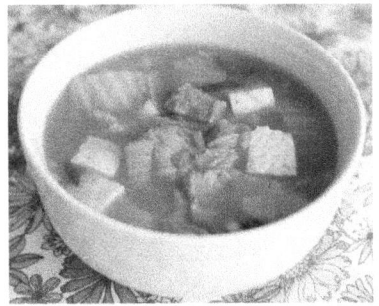

Serves: 6
Time: 3 Hours 10 Minutes
Calories: 110
Protein: 1 Gram
Fat: 12 Grams
Net Carbs: 1.6 Grams
Ingredients:
- 1/2 lb. Pork Belly, Fresh
- Sea Salt & Black Pepper to Taste
- ¾ lb. Napa Cabbage, Chopped
- ½ Cup Spring Onions, Chopped Fine
- ¼ Cup Button Mushrooms
- 1 Teaspoon Stevia Sweetener
- 1 Teaspoon Ground Paprika
- 2 Tablespoons Coconut Aminos
- 3 Tablespoons Sesame Oil
- 4 Cups Water

Directions:
1. Start by cutting your pork belly into strips, and season with salt and pepper.
2. get out your slow cooker, and add in your mushrooms, spring onions and cabbage.
3. Get out a small bowl and mix together your stevia, sesame oil, water, coconut aminos and paprika.
4. Pour this mixture into your slow cooker over your meat and vegetables and cook on high for three hours. Adjust your seasoning as needed and serve warm.

Broccoli & Bacon Casserole

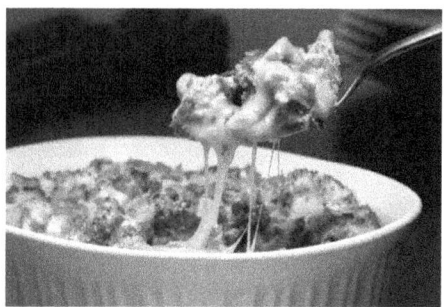

Serves: 4
Time: 50 Minutes
Calories: 325
Protein: 22 Grams
Fat: 24 Grams
Net Carbs: 4.8 Grams

Ingredients:
- 1 Tablespoon Olive oil
- 2 Cups Broccoli Florets, Cooked
- 8 Eggs
- ¼ Cup Water
- 1 Cup Cottage Cheese
- 1 Teaspoon Thyme, fresh & Chopped
- Sea Salt & Black Pepper to Taste
- 3 Ounces Bacon, Crumbled
- 2 Tablespoons Feta Cheese, Crumbled

Directions:
1. Start by heating your oven to 380, and then get out a casserole dish. Coat it with your olive oil, and put your broccoli on the bottom, sprinkling with salt and pepper. Add your cottage cheese and thyme next.
2. Get out a bowl and whisk your eggs with ¼ cup of water, seasoning with salt and pepper. Pour your egg mixture in next, and then add in your crumbled feta and bacon. Cook for thirty-five minutes.
3. Allow it to rest for ten minutes before slicing to serve warm.

Bacon & Spinach Casserole

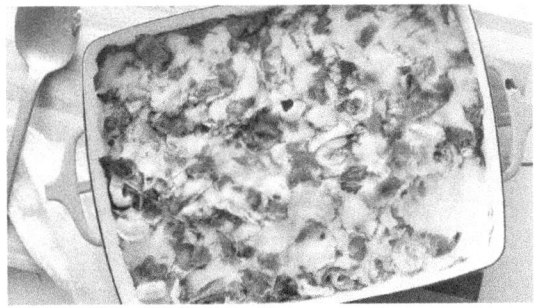

Serves: 5
Time: 30 Minutes
Calories: 502
Protein: 27 Grams
Fat: 42 Grams
Net Carbs: 3 Grams

Ingredients:
- 1 Teaspoon Tallow
- 8 Slices Bacon
- 8 Eggs
- ¾ lb. Spinach, Fresh & Chopped
- Sea Salt & Black Pepper to Taste
- 1 Cup Parmesan Cheese

Directions:
1. Start by heating your oven to 400, and then grease your casserole dish with tallow.
2. Lay your bacon on the bottom, and then sprinkle your chopped spinach over your bacon before sprinkling with sea salt.
3. Get out a bowl and whisk your eggs and parmesan together, seasoning with salt and pepper. Pour this mixture in over your spinach.
4. Cook for twenty minutes, and then turn off the oven leaving your casserole dish inside. Allow it to sit for ten to fifteen minutes. The remaining heat will finish cooking your dish.
5. Slice and serve warm.

Buttery Herb Pork Chops

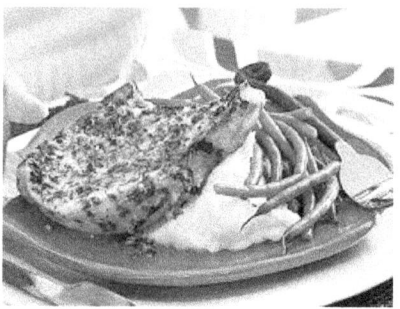

Serves: 2
Time: 30 Minutes
Calories: 333
Protein: 31 Grams
Fat: 23 Grams
Net Carbs: 0 Grams

Ingredients:
- 1 Tablespoon Butter + Enough for Coating
- Sea Salt & Black Pepper to Taste
- 2 Pork Chops, Boneless
- 1 Tablespoon Italian Seasoning
- 1 Tablespoon Italian Parsley, Fresh & Chopped
- 1 Tablespoon Olive Oil

Directions:
1. Start by heating your oven to 350, and then get out a baking dish that's big enough to hold your pork chops. Coat your baking dish with butter.
2. Pat your pork chops dry using a paper towel, placing them into your baking dish and seasoning with Italian seasoning, salt and pepper.
3. Top with parsley, and drizzle with olive oil. Add in ½ a tablespoon of butter on top of each pork chop, and then bake for twenty to twenty-five minutes. Keep in mind that thinner pork chops may cook faster.
4. Serve warm with the juices spooned over the meat.

Parmesan Pork Chops & Asparagus

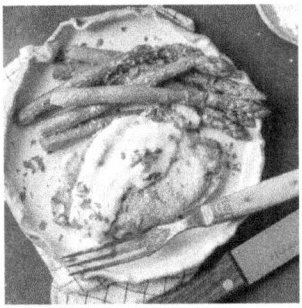

Serves: 2
Time: 35 Minutes
Calories: 370
Protein: 40 Grams
Fat: 21 Grams
Net Carbs: 4 Grams
Ingredients:
- ¼ Cup Parmesan Cheese, Grated
- ¼ Cup Pork Rinds, Crushed
- 1 Teaspoon Garlic Powder
- 2 Pork Chops, Boneless
- Sea Salt & Black Pepper to Taste
- Olive Oil for Drizzling
- ½ lb. Asparagus, Trimmed

Directions:
1. Start by heating your oven to 350, and then get out a baking sheet. In your baking sheet with foil, and then take out a medium bowl.
2. In your bowl mix your parmesan, pork rinds and garlic together.
3. Pat down your pork chops, and then season with salt and pepper.
4. Put your pork chops in the bowl with your pork rind mixture, making sure that it's coated. This will form a "breading". Place them on the baking sheet, and then drizzle oil over each one. Make sure that you don't drench them or the coating won't stay on.
5. Arrange your asparagus around your pork chops on the baking sheet, and then drizzle with olive oil. Season with your asparagus with salt, pepper, and the remaining pork rind mixture.
6. bake for twenty to twenty-five minutes. Keep in mind that thinner pork chops will cook faster. Serve warm.

Sesame Pork with Green Beans

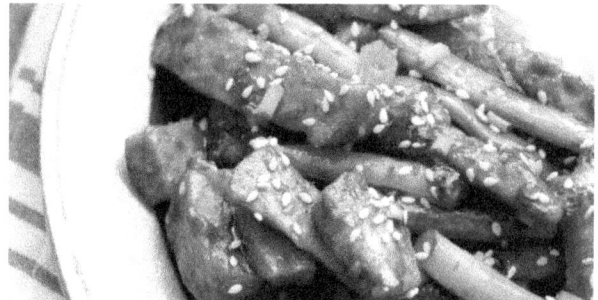

Serves: 2
Time: 15 Minutes
Calories: 366
Protein: 33 Grams
Fat: 24 Grams
Net Carbs: 3 Grams

Ingredients:
- 2 Tablespoons Soy Sauce
- sea Salt & Black Pepper to Taste
- 2 Tablespoons Soy Sauce
- 2 Tablespoons Toasted Sesame Oil, Divided
- 1 Teaspoon Sriracha Sauce
- 1 Cup Green Beans, Fresh

Directions:
1. Get out a cutting board and pat your pork chops dry using a paper towel. Slice your pork chops into thin strips before seasoning with salt and pepper.
2. Get out a large skillet and place it over medium heat with tablespoon of sesame oil. Add in your pork strips, cooking for seven minutes. You will need to stir occasionally to keep your pork strips from burning.
3. Get out a small bowl and combine your remaining tablespoon of sesame oil, soy sauce and Sriracha sauce together. Pour this mixture into the skillet with your pork slices.
4. Add in your green beans before reducing the heat to medium-low. Allow it to simmer for three to five minutes. Divide between bowls before serving warm.

Kalua Pork & Cabbage

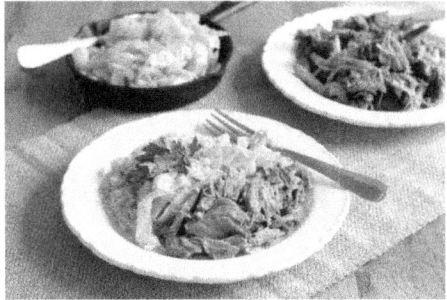

Serves: 2
Time: 8 Hour 10 Minutes
Calories: 550
Protein: 39 Grams
Fat: 41 Grams
Net Carbs: 5 Grams

Ingredients:
- 1 lb. Pork Butt Roast, Boneless
- Sea Salt & Black Pepper to Taste
- 1 Tablespoon Smoked Paprika
- ½ Head Cabbage, Chopped
- ½ Cup Water

Directions:
1. Start by preheating your slow cooker, and season your pork roast with smoked paprika, salt and pepper.
2. Place your roast in your slow cooker, and add in your water. Cook for seven hours, and then transfer it to a plate. Chop your cabbage, placing it in the bottom of your slow cooker with your pork roast on top. Cover, cooking for another hour.
3. Remove your pork roast and then place it on a baking sheet, and then shred it using two forks. Serve the pork with your cooked cabbage.

Blue Cheese Pork Chops

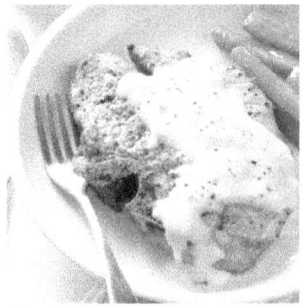

Serves: 2
Time: 15 Minutes
Calories: 669
Protein: 41 Grams
Fat: 34 Grams
Net Carbs: 4 Grams

Ingredients:
- 2 Pork Chops, Boneless
- Sea Salt & Black Pepper to Taste
- 2 Tablespoons Butter
- 1/3 Cup Heavy Whipping Cream
- 1/3 Cup Sour Cream
- 1/3 Cup Blue Cheese Crumbles

Directions:
1. Start by patting your pork chops dry using paper towels before seasoning with salt and pepper. Get out a medium skillet before placing it over medium heat, and then melt your butter. Once it' shot and shimmering, add in your pork chops, and sear for three minutes per side.
2. Transfer your pork chops to a plate, allowing it to rest for three to five minutes, and then get out a medium saucepan. Place your saucepan over medium heat, and melt your blue cheese crumbles. You'll need to stir frequently to make sure that they don't burn. Add the cream and sour cream to the pan. Allow it all to simmer for a few minutes, but make sure to stir occasionally.
3. Add in your pan juice from your pork chops to your cheese mixture, and then allow it to simmer together until thick and creamy.
4. Plate your pork chops with your sauce over them, and serve warm.

Pork Nachos

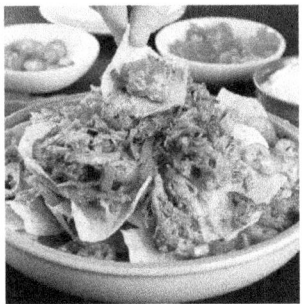

Serves: 2
Time: 15 Minutes
Calories: 587
Protein: 51 Grams
Fat: 51 Grams
Net Carbs: 5 Grams

Ingredients:
- 2 Cups Pork Rinds, Spicy
- 1 Tablespoon Olive Oil + More for Coating
- ½ Cup Mexican Blend Cheese, Shredded
- 1 Cup Carnitas
- 1 Avocado, Diced
- 2 Tablespoons Sour Cream

Directions:
1. Start by heating your oven to 350, and then get out a nine by thirteen inch baking dish.
2. Grease your dish with olive oil, and then put your pork rinds in it. Top with cheese, and bake for five minutes. Transfer this to a cooling rack, allowing it to rest for five minutes.
3. get out a medium skillet, placing it over high heat. Heat up your olive oil, placing your carnitas in the skillet, and then add some pan juices in, cooking until they are crisp. Flip them, and cook briefly on the other side. Divide your pork rinds and cheese between places, and top with carnitas, diced avocado and sour cream. Serve warm.

Pork Burgers & Sriracha Mayonnaise

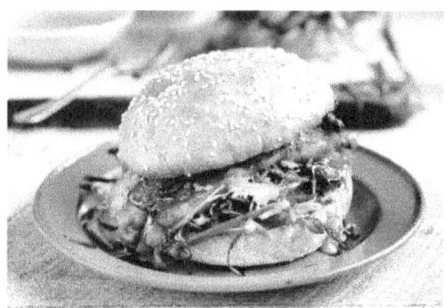

Serves: 2
Time: 20 Minutes
Calories: 575
Protein: 31 Grams
Fat: 49 Grams
Net Carbs: 1 Gram
Ingredients:
- 12 Ounces Ground Pork
- 1 Tablespoon Toasted Sesame Oil
- 2 Scallions, Sliced Thin
- Sea Salt & Black Pepper to Taste
- 1 Tablespoon Sriracha Sauce
- 2 Tablespoons Mayonnaise
- 1 Tablespoon Ghee

Directions:
1. Start by getting out a large bowl and combine your sesame oil, scallions and ground pork together. Season with salt and pepper, and then form two burgers. Make sure to create a dent in each so that your pork will heat evenly and cook all the way through.
2. Get out a large skillet, placing it over medium-high heat, and then heat up your ghee. Your ghee should be shimmering before your add in your patties. Cook for four minutes per side.
3. Get out a small bowl and mix your Sriracha sauce with your mayonnaise, making sure that it's well combined.
4. Transfer your burgers to a plate, allowing them to cool for five minutes before topping with your sauce to serve.

Side Dish Recipes
Cheesy Asparagus

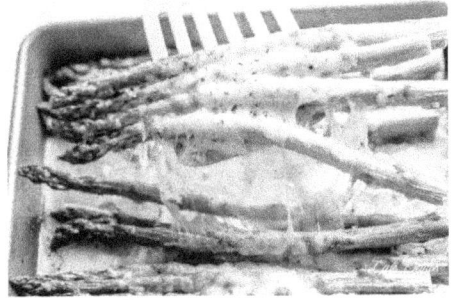

Serves: 2
Time: 20 Minutes
Calories: 253
Protein: 12 Grams
Fat: 21 Grams
Net Carbs: 3 Grams

Ingredients:
- 1 Bunch Asparagus
- 2 Tablespoons Olive Oil
- ½ Cup Parmesan, Grated
- ½ Teaspoon Garlic Powder
- ¼ Cup Pork Rind Crumbs
- Sea Salt & Black Pepper to Taste

Directions:
1. Start by heating your oven to 425.
2. Trim your asparagus, and then get out larger zipper top bag, and then throw in your asparagus and olive oil. Shake well, and then add in your pork rinds, parmesan cheese, and garlic powder. Season with salt and pepper. Shake until your asparagus is fully coated, and then arrange it in a single layer on the baking sheet.
3. Cook for eight to ten minutes, and serve warm.

Spicy Cauliflower

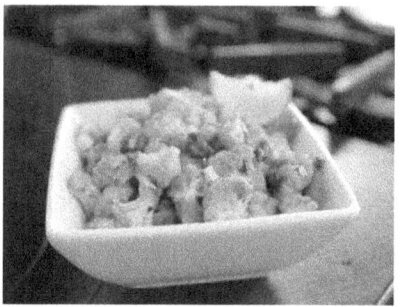

Serves: 2
Time: 35 Minutes
Calories: 145
Protein: 2 Grams
Fat: 13 Grams
Net Carbs: 3 Grams

Ingredients:
- ½ Cauliflower Head, Chopped into Florets
- 1 Tablespoon Olive Oil
- 1 Teaspoon Garlic Powder
- Sea Salt & Black Pepper
- 1 Tablespoon Butter
- ¼ Cup Buffalo Wing Sauce

Directions:
1. Start by preheating your oven to 400, and then get out a baking sheet. Line your baking sheet with parchment paper, and then get out a mixing bowl. Drizzle your cauliflower with olive oil and then season with salt, pepper and garlic powder.
2. Get out a baking sheet, and arrange the cauliflower in a single spread out layer. Roast for fifteen minutes, and then stir well. Cook for ten minutes.
3. Get out a small saucepan and mix your buffalo wing sauce and butter, cooking it over medium heat until it's melted and mixed well.
4. Brush your cauliflower down with the sauce, cooking for five more minutes and serve warm.

Stuffed Mushrooms

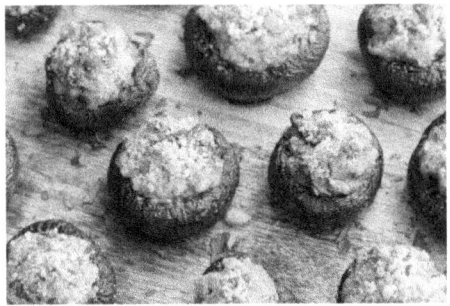

Serves: 2
Time: 25 Minutes
Calories: 139
Protein: 8 Grams
Fat: 10 Grams
Net Carbs: 2 Grams

Ingredients:
- 2 Ounces Lump Crab Meat
- 1 Tablespoon Scallion, Sliced (Green Parts Only)
- ¼ Teaspoon Paprika
- ¼ Teaspoon Onion Powder
- 6-8 Cremini Mushrooms, Stemmed
- 2 Tablespoons Avocado Oil Mayonnaise
- 1 Teaspoon Parsley, Fresh & Chopped
- Sea Salt & Black Pepper to Taste

Directions:
1. Start by heating your oven to 350, and then line a baking sheet with parchment paper. Get out a medium bowl and mix together your scallions, mayonnaise, crab meat, onion powder and paprika together. Mix well and season with salt and pepper.
2. Get out a prepared baking sheet, arranging your mushrooms evenly apart, and make sure the gill side is up. Fill each with a spoonful of your mixture, and then bake for fifteen minutes.
3. garnish with parsley before serving warm.

Lemon Spinach

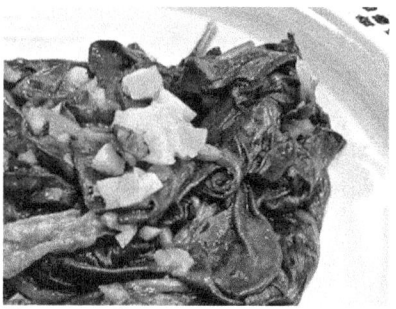

Serves: 2
Time: 10 Minutes
Calories: 82
Protein: 2 Grams
Fat: 7 Grams
Net Carbs: 2 Grams

Ingredients:
- 1 Tablespoon Olive Oil
- 1 Clove Garlic, Minced
- 1 Shallow, Sliced Thin
- 4 Cups Spinach, Fresh
- 1 Tablespoon Capers, Chopped
- ¼ Lemon, Juiced
- Sea Salt & Black Pepper to Taste

Directions:
1. Start by getting out a skillet and heating up your olive oil over medium heat. Add in your garlic once your oil begins to shimmer, and then add in your shallow. Sauté for a minute, and stir continuously so that it doesn't burn.
2. Add in your spinach, capers and lemon juice, cooking for a minute more. Your spinach should wilt, and then season with salt and pepper.
3. Serve topped with lemon zest.

Red Cabbage Salad

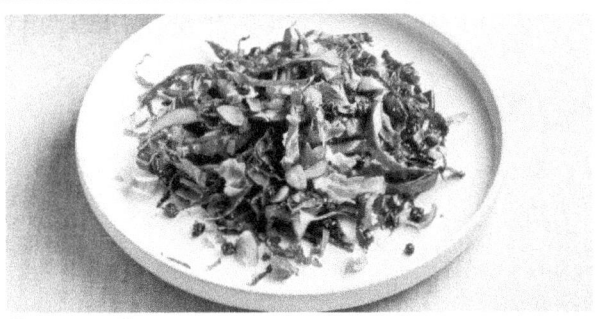

Serves: 6
Time: 15 Minutes
Calories: 200
Protein: 6.3 Grams
Fat: 15.5 Grams
Net Carbs: 2 Grams

Ingredients:
- 2 Cloves Garlic, Sliced Fine
- 1 lb. Red Cabbage, Shredded
- 4 Slices Bacon, Crispy & Crumbled
- ½ Cup Olive Oil
- 2 Tablespoons Lemon Juice, Fresh
- ½ Teaspoon Tarragon
- ½ Teaspoon Mustard Seeds

Directions:
1. Start by rinsing your cabbage, and then place it in a food processor to shred it. Place your shredded cabbage in a bowl before seasoning with salt, pepper, bacon and garlic. Toss until well combined.
2. Get out a small bowl and whisk your tarragon, lemon juice, olive oil and mustard seeds together.
3. Pour this dressing over your cabbage salad, tossing until it's well combined.
4. Serve immediately.

Garlic Mushrooms

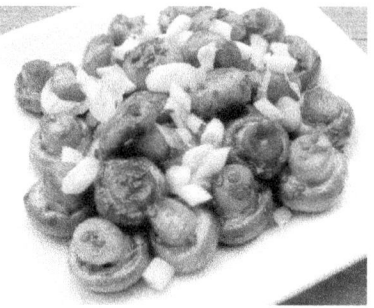

Serves: 8
Time: 1 Hour 5 Minutes
Calories: 40
Protein: 4.5 Grams
Fat: 1 Gram
Net Carbs: 3 Grams
Ingredients:
- 6 Cloves Garlic
- Sea Salt to Taste
- 2 ½ lbs. White Mushrooms, Fresh
- 2 Cups Vinegar, Distilled

Directions:
1. Start by blanching your mushrooms in the vinegar for an hour, making sure that your garlic and salt is in the mixture too. Drain your mushrooms, and then keep them refrigerated. Serve on the side of any main dish.

Braised Lemon Mushrooms

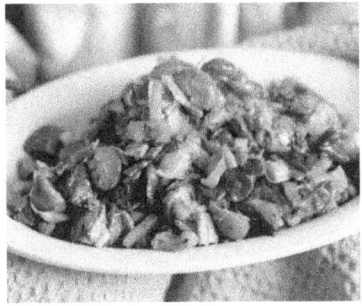

Serves: 4
Time: 20 Minutes
Calories: 100
Protein: 3.7 Grams
Fat: 8 Grams
Net Carbs: 4 Grams

Ingredients:
- 2 Tablespoons Olive Oil
- 1 Teaspoon Butter
- 1 Clove Garlic, Grated
- 1 Lemon, Juiced
- 1 lb. Mushrooms, Fresh & Halved
- 1 Teaspoon Lemon Zest
- 1 Tablespoon Thyme, Fresh & Chopped
- Sea Salt & Black Pepper to Taste

Directions:
1. Heat your butter and oil in a large frying pan before adding in your mushrooms. Cook for three minutes. Do not stir.
2. Stir in your mushrooms, cooking for five to six minutes more. Add in your lemon zest and garlic, cooking for another minute. It should become fragrant and your garlic should be lightly browned.
3. Season your mushrooms with salt, pepper and thyme. Drizzle with lemon juice, and stir well. Serve warm.

Conclusion

Now you know everything you need to get started on healthy ketogenic dinners that will keep to your lifestyle and fitness goals without breaking the bank or leave your stomach growling. Remember that just because you've gone keto doesn't mean that you should go hungry! Always treat yourself to new recipes to keep it interesting, and just pick a recipe to get started working your way down the list. Go meatless occasionally for the extra health benefits and boost to your budget too!

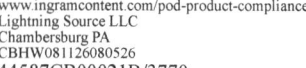
www.ingramcontent.com/pod-product-compliance
Lightning Source LLC
Chambersburg PA
CBHW081126080526
44587CB00021B/3770